Understanding Diabetes "Type 2"

R Young Rev 6

Richard Young Bio:
https://amzn.to/44Cciqf

Understanding Diabetes:

The Author was diagnosed with Type 2
Diabetes in 2005 and still kicking 20 years
later.

This Guide is a collection of knowledge gained
by researching type 2 and converting medical
terms into plain English which should make a
more understandable read.

Take for instance the term "Type 2 Diabetes", it
is also described as "Late or Adult-onset
Diabetes", "Non-Insulin-Dependent Diabetes"
or now it is called "**Diabetes mellitus type
2**". Not any name truly describes how sneaky
and deadly this destructive condition can be,
and most do not know they have diabetes.

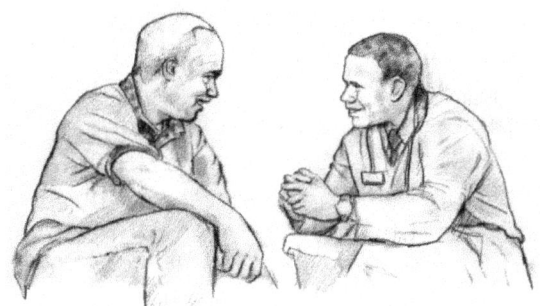

New to Diabetes?

Don't feel alone, there were 1,699 other people who got the news the same day as you.

This book is a Guide for the "Newly Diagnosed Diabetes Patient" and a way to organize and make sense out of all the sometimes-confusing data.

If the doctor that told you about your diabetes gave you this book, he or she would do you a great favor. You will now have a better understanding of diabetes, and you can go over and over the material until you feel comfortable.

My goal for the book is to make all the technical "Doctor Speak" into something the average guy can understand. It was only after my first visit that I started to have some questions about what my doctor was trying to say. I hope that this guide will answer those questions that pop up.

Today we are a nation obsessed with fast food and lack of activity. I have a lifestyle that sets me behind a computer screen working for too long and then I rest by watching TV.

The research for this guide includes chapters on having a nutritious diet with recipes for great meals and recommendations for exercise programs.

Startling results on who has diabetes and who **will have diabetes** are contained in these pages. OK, here are some background stats.

All Diabetes Cases 2003:

- **1,700 New cases** of Diabetes Diagnosed Every Day in the US.
- **150,000 People Die** every year from Diabetes.
- **16,000,000 People** that Now Have Diabetes.

Costs in My small state:

- $832,000,000 in medical expenses each year.
- $460,000 in lost productivity.
- National Costs between $174 Billion and 218 billion each year.

Television & Diabetes

No one ever said when I was growing up that "Fast Food" is bad for you, on the contrary, watching all those commercials on the TV, it always said how great and convenient all that stuff was. NOW, after listening to the claims of company's selling food on TV, I cannot understand how they get away with what they say. Let the brainwashing begin, and TV shows are the best. How many times did you ask your mom for something you saw on TV as a kid?

From someone who knows Commercial TV (over 40 years in the business), I now live by these four rules:

- Rule 1: Never believe any TV commercial about food.
- Rule 2: Fast Food is rarely good for you.
- Rule 3: Portion size is always way too much for a healthy lifestyle.
- Rule 4: See Rule 1.

At about the time that middle age starts to turn into older age, without warning diabetes starts to take hold for too many of us. This is when you start having blood sugar problems, but there are no symptoms. Looking back, I think that I had Diabetes say 5 years before diagnosed. Those 5 years gave it a head start on what will be a fight for the rest of my life.

Confused?

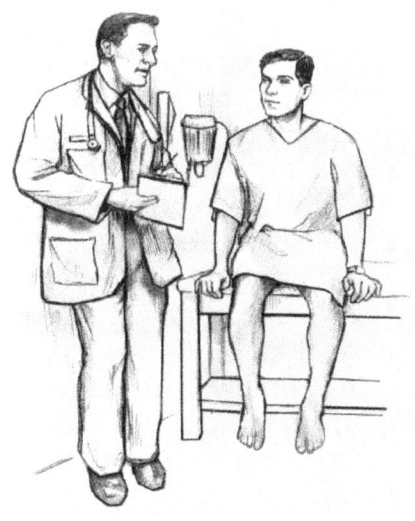

Do I have Diabetes?

The questions in this chapter of the book represent a sample of people who had, or were developing, Type 2 diabetes, and to me they show a lack of knowledge about diabetes.

The questions show real questions, some are about life and death problems. Material in this book should answer all these questions.

- What's the average blood pressure for a patient with diabetes type 2??? When it's considered high?? is 168/88 life threatening???
- I have checked (blood glucose) often now and if I don't eat for a couple of hours, I get low. Could this be the beginning of diabetes like my pancreas is going out of whack?? Help please!!!!
- In early January I went for my physical and I had type 2 diabetes. I was the youngest patient that my doctor ever had to diagnose this condition. I weighed 200 and my blood sugar was 232. So far, I have lost 19 pounds. I totally changed my lifestyle and I'm exercising every day. If I keep this up, will I be able to get rid of my type 2?
- Can losing weight recover from type 2 diabetes?
- I have low blood sugar but recently I looked up symptoms of diabetes and I have: Blurry Vision Fatigue Irritation Increase hunger—-Even if I don't have diabetes how does it explain my blurry vision? Can low blood sugar lead to diabetes?
- Can years of hypertension cause diabetes?

- My husband has type 2 diabetes and it seems like no matter what he raises his blood sugar above the roof. I mean like snacks and dinner type foods and what about lunch meat? Do I need to avoid the whites such as sugar white flour white rice potatoes Etc. In other words, do you eat meat with feathers or fins?
- Does anybody know any recipes suitable for people with diabetes?
- Does taking Prozac make a diabetic's blood-sugar hard to control?
- Is Ginkgo Balboa safe?
- I need help on when to do blood tests.
- How bad is type 2 diabetes?
- How does diabetes cause people to lose their feet?
- How does Diabetes hurt the skin? What are the signs of Diabetes?
- How many carbs should I take and I'm diabetes type 2?
- Is there a limit on how much alcohol you can drink? I am now drinking 3 or 5 pints every Saturday night.
- I was feeling really bad and I checked my blood sugar. It read 406 so I drank all kinds of water and took my pills before I went to bed. The reading was 389. This morning it was 291. What do you do to get the reading down?

These are just a few of the hundreds of questions I found on the web, did you hear your question?

It shows that even with doctor's instructions, a new patient will not understand all the instructions.

What is Diabetes Type 2

Diabetes type 2 (90% of all cases) is a metabolic disorder that is characterized by high blood glucose in the context of insulin resistance in any age group, and they are getting younger and younger – sadly!

Type 2 contrasts with diabetes mellitus type 1, where type 1 is an absolute insulin deficiency due to destruction of beta islet cells in the pancreas.

The classic symptoms of diabetes are excess thirst, frequent urination, and constant hunger.

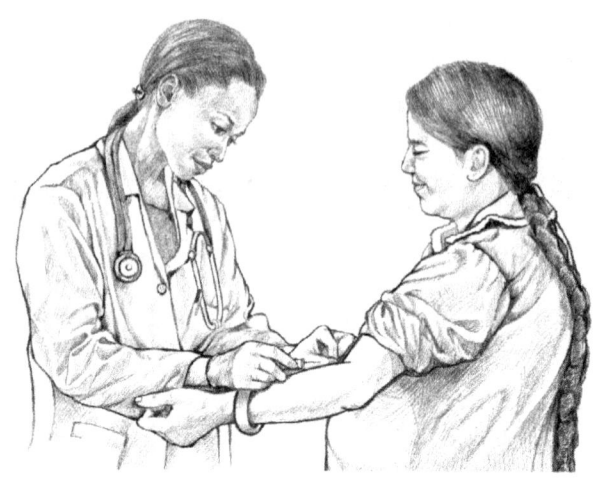

Blood Screenings

In 2010 it was estimated that 285 million people globally had diabetes. Of the total, type 2 diabetes makes up about 90% of cases and the other 10% due primarily to diabetes mellitus type 1 and gestational diabetes of pregnant women. Over 23.6 million children and adults in the United States – 7.8% of the population have diabetes.

There are 57 million people who have pre-diabetes, and 1.6 million cases of diabetes are diagnosed in people aged 20 years or older each year.

Women seem to be at a greater risk as do certain ethnic groups, such as South Asians, Pacific Islanders, Latinos, and Native Americans.

Traditionally considered a disease of adults, type 2 diabetes is increasingly diagnosed in children in parallel with rising obesity rates. There have been correlations between the increase of processed foods from the 1950's and the explosion of diabetes during the same period.

Type 2 diabetes is now diagnosed as often as type 1 diabetes in teenagers in the United States. Obesity is thought to be the primary cause of type 2 diabetes in people who are genetically predisposed to the disease.

Type 2 diabetes Management:

Jogging and Exercise

Type 2 diabetes is initially managed by increasing exercise and dietary modification. If blood glucose levels are not adequately lowered by these measures, medications such as Metformin working up to insulin may be needed. Blood sugar levels should be checked by all with diabetes routinely.

Diabetes have increased markedly over the last 50 years in parallel with obesity. As of 2012, there are about 285 million people with the disease compared to around 30 million in 1985. Long-term complications from high blood sugar can include heart disease, strokes, diabetic retinopathy where eyesight is affected, kidney failure which may need dialysis, and poor circulation of limbs leading to amputations.

The nasty thing about type 2 is that until diagnosed the person is usually not aware they have the disorder. I know that after the doctor first talks about diabetes the patient may not give the diagnosis its due regard due to not feeling sick.

In my case I originally was on Metformin but did not feel that I needed to strictly follow the daily dosage because there were no effects by missing doses.

History of Diabetes:

Diabetes is one of the first diseases described in an Egyptian manuscript from c. 1500 BCE mentioning **"too great emptying of the urine.** "The first described cases are believed to be of type 1 diabetes. Indian physicians around the same time identified the disease and classified it as 'Madhumeha" or honey urine noting that the urine would attract ants.

The term **"Diabetes"** or **"to pass through"** was first used in 230 BCE by the Greek Apollonius of Memphis. The disease was rare during the time of the Roman empire with Galen commenting that he had only seen two cases during his career.*

Type 1 and type 2 diabetes were identified as separate conditions for the first time by the Indian physicians Sushruta and Charaka in 400-500 AD with type 1 associated with youth and type 2 with being overweight.

The term **"mellitus"** or **"from honey"** was added by the Briton John Rolle in the late 1700's to separate the condition from diabetes insipidus which is also associated with frequent urination.

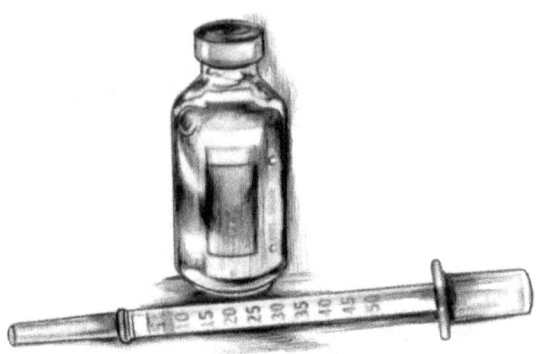

Effective treatment was not developed until the early part of the 20th century when the Canadians Frederick Banting and Charles Best discovered insulin in 1921 and 1922. This was followed by the development of the long acting NPH insulin in the 1940s.

*This Author's hypothesis about the "Rare" condition before 1900 and the discovery of insulin:
Most type 1 cases of children probably died before reaching adulthood keeping the genetic passing of type 1 diabetes to a minimum. Before 1900 the life expectancy was less than 50 years, so type 2 cases rarely happened because of the exercise and natural diet at the time and complications of untreated type 2 diabetes may have been considered death by old.

The Signs and Symptoms:

The classic symptoms of diabetes are:
Polyuria (frequent urination)
Polydipsia (increased thirst)
Polyphagia (increased hunger)
Weight loss (most would be happy with this one)
Pain or numbness in the feet or hands.

Other symptoms that are commonly present at diagnosis include:
History of blurred vision (I needed new set of glasses every 3 months)
Itchiness (Uncontrolled need to Scratch – Been there done that*)
Peripheral neuropathy (Nerve damage)
Recurrent vaginal infections
Fatigue (Getting older everyone tends to slow down; this could seem natural)

Many people, however, have no symptoms during the first few years and are diagnosed only during routine testing.
People with type 2 diabetes mellitus rarely present with nonketotic hyperosmolar **coma** (a condition of very high blood sugar associated with a decreased level of consciousness and low blood pressure).

*Uncontrollable Itch; I have found that itching can be controlled when it first starts by applying Halobetasol propionate 0.05% (generic name), also called Ultravate (patented name) an ultra-highly potent topical steroid, to the area and then managing to keep your hands from itching the area for 20 min.

Usually this happens to me at bedtime and after 20 min the itch goes away, and I am asleep. This ointment falls in the class **Very potent:** it is said up to 600 times stronger than over the counter hydrocortisone. Needless to say, this stuff is a fantastic drug to have around and is normally used to treat **eczema and skin conditions.**

My doctor has used the combination of Kenalog (injection) along with a Prednisone (pills) that work wonders if my eczema itching gets out of control. I may have that combination once a year when needed. Also, it is best to keep your fingernails trimmed back so you will not scratch your skin while asleep due to the slow healing with Diabetes.

However, Kenalog & Prednisone **will** increase glucose levels for a short time.

Complications of Type 2 Diabetes:

Type 2 diabetes is typically a chronic disease associated with a **ten-year-shorter life** expectancy. This is partly due to a number of complications with which diabetes is associated.

- Two to four times the risk of **cardiovascular disease** (Venous & Arterial blood veins)
- Ischemic **heart disease and stroke** (Reduce blood to the heart and Brain)
- **Lower limb amputations; 20-fold increase** (Surgery)
- **Frequent infections** & Increased rates of hospitalizations.

In the developed world, and increasingly elsewhere, type 2 diabetes is the largest cause of:

- **Non-traumatic blindness** (loss of sight)
- **Kidney failure**
- It has also been associated with an increased risk of cognitive dysfunction and **dementia** (Brain disorder) through

disease processes such as **Alzheimer's disease** and **vascular dementia**.

- **Nigricans Acanthosis** (brown to black spots on the skin)
- **Sexual dysfunction** (Erectile Dysfunction)

Author: All of these complications of type 2 diabetes are scary and life changing events. Although you cannot cure type 2 at this time, you sure can follow the recommendations and tips in the following chapters to make your life better and live longer.

BMI, Lifestyle and Genetic Factors:

To find BMI: Multiply body weight in pounds by 703. Divide that number by height in inches. Divide that number by height in inches again. Find the resulting number below.

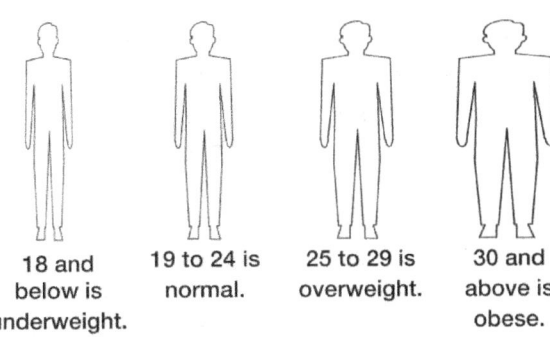

18 and below is underweight.

19 to 24 is normal.

25 to 29 is overweight.

30 and above is obese.

BMI

Even a lack of sleep has been linked to type 2 diabetes. This is believed to act through sleeps effect on metabolism.

The nutritional status of a mother during fetal development may also play a role, with one proposed mechanism being that of altered DNA methylation.

Lifestyle:

While some causes are under personal control, such as diet and obesity, others, such as increasing age, female gender, and genetics, is not. A number of lifestyle factors are known to be important:

- **Obesity** (defined by a **B**ody **M**ass **I**ndex of greater than thirty)
- **Lack of physical activity**, poor diet, stress, and urbanization are believed to cause 7% of cases.
- **Excess body fat** is associated with 30% of cases in those of Chinese and Japanese descent, 60-80% of cases in those of European and African descent, and 100% of Pima American Indians and Pacific Islanders.
- **High waist–hip ratio** for those who are not obese.
- **Consumption of sugar-sweetened drinks in EXCESS** is associated with an increased risk. (So much for the Pepsi and Coke drinkers, learn to like non-sweetened drinks)
- **The type of fats in the diet** are also important.
- Saturated fats and Trans fatty acids (found in **processed food**) increasing the risk of coronary heart disease by raising LDL (Bad cholesterol).

- Polyunsaturated and monounsaturated fat (found in **natural foods**) raise HDL (Good cholesterol), decrease the risk of cardiovascular disease and may be protective against insulin resistance (main cause of type 2 diabetes).

Data from the landmark Framingham Heart Study showed that, for a given level of LDL, the risk of heart disease increases 10-fold as the HDL varies from high to low. On the converse, however, for a fixed level of HDL, the risk increases 3-fold as LDL varies from low to high. Even people with very low LDL levels are exposed to increased risk if their HDL levels are not high enough.

Healthy Eating Plan Helps You Learn About Nutrition

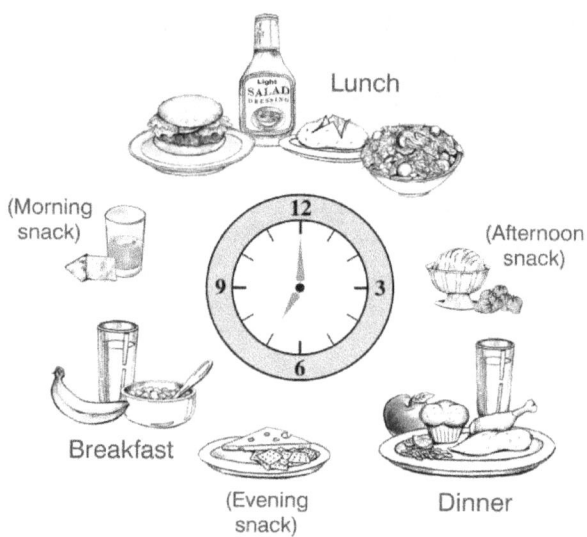

Losing weight is not just about looking good in a pair of jeans; it's also about improving your overall health. Diets that suggest you drink only liquids or eliminate carbohydrates or fats are hogwash. Our bodies are fueled by the nutrients in the foods we eat. Any diet that requires you to cut some of the most important foods can ruin your health.

Poor nutritional health contributes to diabetes, heart disease, osteoporosis, cancer, and other life altering health conditions. Most of the foods marketed by manufacturers as "healthy" aren't healthy at all. Nope. Not even a bit.

If you don't know what to look for, it's easy to believe that frozen dinners, nutritional shakes, snack bars and other processed foods are alright to eat. When you opt for a healthy eating plan instead of a "diet," you learn to make every calorie count by choosing foods that give you the best nutritional bang for your efforts.

Genetics

As of 2011, more than **36 genes** have been found that contribute to the risk of type 2 diabetes. All of these genes together still only account for 10% of the total inheritable part of the disease.

Most cases of diabetes involve many genes, with each being a small contributor to an increased chance of becoming a type 2 diabetic. If one identical twin has diabetes, the chance of the other developing diabetes within his lifetime is greater than 90% while the rate for non-identical siblings is 25-50%.

Predisposed to diabetes

Increased diabetes risk for users of these medications:

- **Glucocorticoids** (cell metabolism of glucose
- **Thiazides** (often used to treat high blood pressure)
- **Beta blockers** (used for irregular heartbeat & the management of cardiac arrhythmias)
- **Atypical anti-psychotics** (group of antipsychotic tranquilizing)
- **Statins** (used to lower cholesterol levels).
- Those women who have previously had gestational diabetes are at a higher risk of developing type 2 diabetes.

Other health problems associated include:

- **Acromegaly** (results when the anterior pituitary gland produces excess growth hormone)
- **Cushing's Syndrome** (caused by taking glucocorticoid drugs, or diseases that result in excess cortisol)
- **Hyperthyroidism** (overactive thyroid')
- **Pheochromocytoma** (Brain tumor)
- **Certain cancers** such as glucagonomas (Very rare tumor of the alpha cells of the pancreas)
- **Testosterone deficiency** ("Low T" in men) is also associated with type 2 diabetes.

Blood Testing for Type 2:

Please check the chapter on drugs that will raise meter reading before testing.

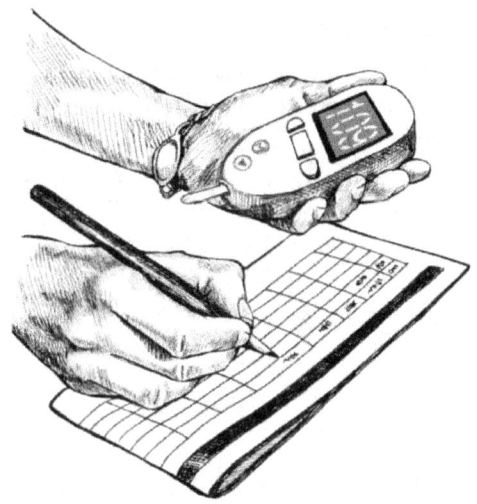

Logging meter readings

Normal Condition:

When you wake up in the morning and before breakfast.

- "Fasting Glucose" should be less than 110 mg/dl.
- Before a meal between 70 and 150 mg/dl.
- Less than 180 mg/dL after meals

- Before bed the range is between 110 and 150 mg/dl.

Abnormal Low Blood Glucose:

If blood glucose readings are **below 70** mg/dl, eat one tablespoon of sugar, honey, or maple syrup, two tablespoons of raisins, three or four glucose tablets, or drink one-half cup of juice or regular soda. Wait 15 minutes and take the reading again. If blood sugar levels are above 180 mg/dl, walk around for 10 or 15 minutes and take the reading again. I know that low blood sugar can be very bad because both brain and body will tell you to do something quick to get it back to above 50!

Abnormal High Condition:

A fasting blood glucose level of 126 mg/dL and higher most often means you have diabetes. For type 2 diabetics who are non-insulin, exercise and diet are the best tools. Blood glucose monitoring is, in that case, simply a tool to evaluate the success of diet and exercise.

THE CBM:

I now use a CBM: Constant Blood Monitor. My CBM is a two-device unit that records my Blood Sugars all day 24 hours each day for ~ 14 days without changing units. My units are **Abbott Freestyle Libre 3 Plus** sensor and display, with alarm if numbers get too **Hi or Low, recommend, ask Dr.**

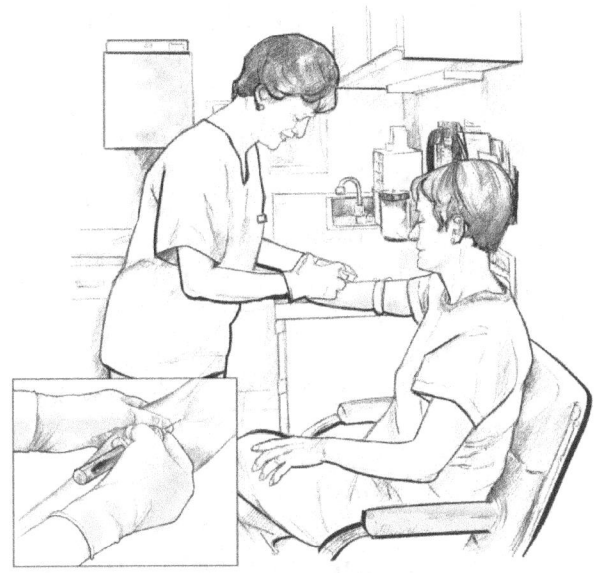

HgA1c Testing

HgA1c

The National Health Institute Recommendation:

Your health care provider may suspect that you have diabetes if your blood sugar level is higher than 200 mg/dL. To confirm the diagnosis, one or more of the following tests must be done.

Diabetes blood tests:

- Fasting blood glucose level — diabetes is diagnosed if it is higher than 126 mg/dL two times
- Hemoglobin A1c test–
    - Normal: Less than 5.7%
    - Pre-diabetes: 5.7% – 6.4%
    - Diabetes: 6.5% or higher
- Oral glucose tolerance test — diabetes is diagnosed if glucose level is higher than 200 mg/dL after 2 hours

Diabetes screening is recommended for:

- Overweight children who have other risk factors for diabetes, starting at age 10 and repeated every 2 years
- Overweight adults (BMI greater than 25) who have other risk factors
- Adults over age 45 every 3 years

You should see your health care provider every 3 months. At these visits, you can expect your health care provider to:

- Check your blood pressure
- Check the skin and bones on your feet and legs
- Check to see if your feet are becoming numb
- Examine the back part of the eye with a special lighted instrument called an ophthalmoscope

The following tests will help you and your doctor monitor your diabetes and prevent problems:

- Have your blood pressure checked at least every year (blood pressure goals should be 130/80 mm/Hg or lower).
- Have your hemoglobin A1C test (HbA1c) every 6 months if your diabetes is well controlled; otherwise, every 3 months.
- Have your cholesterol and triglyceride levels checked yearly (aim for LDL levels below 70-100 mg/dL).
- Get yearly tests to make sure your kidneys are working well (microalbuminuria and serum creatinine).
- Visit your eye doctor at least once a year, or more often if you have signs of diabetic eye disease.
- See the dentist every 6 months for a thorough dental cleaning and exam. Make sure your dentist and hygienist know that you have diabetes.

Note from the Author:

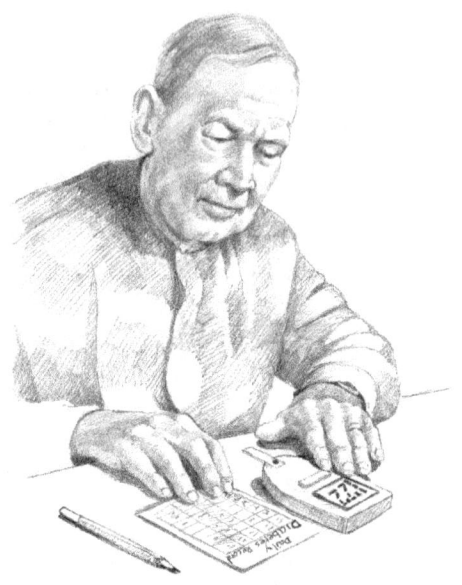

Normally you take your **"before meal"** reading and then another one **"2 hours later"**. The comparison of before and after is the key to determining how your diabetic condition is changed by the food you eat. The meter reading and what you ate should be logged into your logbook each time you use the meter. It is true that most meters save a number of readings but the whole thing is for **"You"** and not the doctor.

The doctor already knows you have Diabetes and he or she probably gave you a meter and some test strips to get you started along with a prescription to get a hundred or so more strips. The thing most doctors sometimes forget to pass on to you *is why* you are testing.

The reason why you test is for you to see how different foods affect your system. If for instance you get a 135 before a meal and 2 hours later you get a 185, you will know that what you ate raised your glucose level 50 points even after 2 hours. That is why it is important to log what you have for each meal so that you can compare how different foods affect your system. Then you will know which foods are best for you.

I have a fantastic Doctor, but when I was getting set up for a meter with all the information at once I did not remember why I test but just how to test.

FYI: Doctors are given test meter kits by the companies that make them so you will use their test strips (cost $.50 to over $1.00 each test), so be sure to ask for a kit from your doctor, you should **never** need to buy one at the pharmacy.

Note, you will need to buy a replacement battery for the meter occasionally. My One Touch takes two CR2032 batteries easily found at a drug store. If you use a CBM, the battery is rechargeable in the Monitor.

Drugs and Medication:

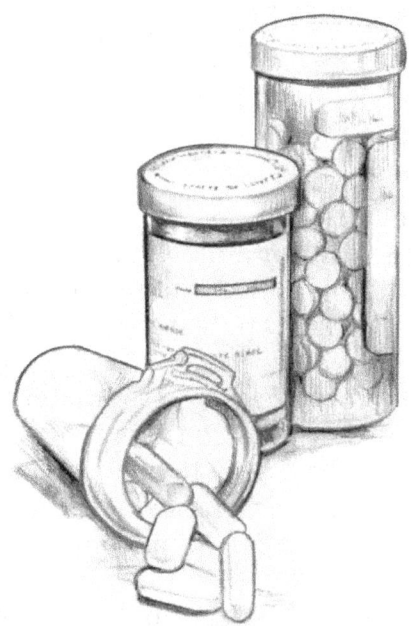

Metformin

There are several classes of anti-diabetic medications available.
Metformin is generally recommended as a

first line treatment as there is some evidence that it *decreases mortality.*

Other classes of medications include sulfonylureas, no sulfonylurea, secretagogues, alpha glucosidase inhibitors, thiazolidinediones, glucagon-like peptide-1 analog, dipeptidyl peptidase-4 inhibitors (sitagliptin or Patent Name Januvia).

Metformin should not be used by those with severe kidney or liver problems. Injections of insulin may either be added to any oral medication or used alone.

Most people do not initially need insulin. When it is used, a long-acting formulation is typically added at night, with oral medications being continued. Doses are then increased to effect (blood sugar levels being well controlled). When nightly insulin is insufficient twice daily insulin may achieve better control.

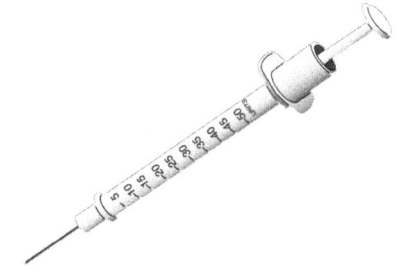

Insulin injections

The long acting insulins, glargine and detemir, do not appear much better than neutral protamine Hagedorn (NPH) insulin but have a significantly greater cost making them, as of 2010, not cost effective.

An insulin pump is an alternative to multiple daily injections of insulin by insulin syringe or an insulin pen and allows for intensive insulin therapy when used in conjunction with blood glucose monitoring and carb counting. In those who are pregnant, insulin is generally the treatment of choice.

Surgery:

Weight loss surgery in those who are obese is an effective measure to treat diabetes. Many are able to maintain normal blood sugar levels with little or no medications following surgery and long-term mortality is decreased.

There is, however, some short-term mortality risk of less than 1% from the surgery. The body mass index cutoffs for when surgery is appropriate are not yet clear. It, however, is recommended that this option be considered in those who are unable to get both their weight and blood sugar under control.

Design a Diet:

From the National Institute of Health:

The Diabetes Food Pyramid, which resembles the old USDA food guide pyramid, splits foods into six groups in a range of serving sizes. In the Diabetes Food Pyramid, food groups are based on carbohydrate and protein content instead of their food classification type. A person with diabetes should eat more of the food at the bottom of the pyramid (grains, beans, vegetables) than those on the top (fats and sweets). This diet will help keep your heart and body systems healthy.

Most people with Type 2 diabetes are overweight.

You can improve blood sugar levels by following a meal plan that has:

- **Fewer calories**
- **Carbohydrates** (less than 55 grams per meal and less than 15 grams for snacks)
- **Healthy monounsaturated fats**

Examples of foods that are high in monounsaturated fats include peanut or almond butter, almonds, and walnuts. You can substitute these foods for carbohydrates but keep portions small because these foods are high in calories. Learn how to read nutrition labels to help you make better food choices.

Often, you can improve type 2 diabetes control by losing weight (about 10% of total body mass) and increasing physical activity (for example, 30 minutes of walking per day). My goal is BMI 19 to 24.

In addition to making lifestyle changes, some people will need to take pills or insulin injections to control their blood sugar.

CHILDREN AND TYPE 2 DIABETES

Children with type 2 diabetes present special challenges. Meal plans should consider the number of calories children need to grow. Kids often need three small meals and three snacks to meet their calories needed. The goal is a healthy weight (most children with type 2 diabetes are obese) and increase physical activity.

Changes in eating habits and increased exercise help improve blood sugar control. When at parties or during holidays, your child may still eat sugary foods. But during other times of the day, the child should have fewer carbohydrates.

Children who eat birthday cake, Halloween candy, or other sweets should NOT have the usual daily number of potatoes, pasta, or rice. This substitution helps keep calories and carbohydrates in better balance.

MEAL PLANNING

One of the most challenging aspects of managing diabetes is meal planning. Work closely with the doctor and dietitian to design a meal plan that keeps the blood sugar (glucose) levels near normal. The meal plan should give you or your child the proper number of calories to maintain a healthy body weight.

Doesn't mean you or your child must completely give up any food, but it does change the kinds of foods your child should eat routinely. Choose foods with moderate amounts of carbohydrates (about 30 – 45 grams per meal) to help keep blood sugar levels under good control. Foods should also provide enough calories to maintain a healthy weight. Regular monitoring of blood sugar (glucose) at home will help you learn how different foods affect blood sugar (glucose) levels.

Recommendations:

A registered dietitian can help you decide how to balance the carbohydrates, protein, and fat in your diet. Here are some general guidelines:

The amount of each type of food you eat depends on:

- **Your diet**
- **Your weight**
- **How often do you exercise**
- **Your other health risks**

Everyone has individual needs. Work with your doctor, and possibly a dietitian, to develop a meal plan that works for you.

The Diabetes Food Pyramid, which resembles the old USDA food guide pyramid, splits foods into six groups in a range of serving sizes. In the Diabetes Food Pyramid, food groups are based on carbohydrate and protein content instead of their food type. A person with diabetes should eat more of the foods at the bottom of the pyramid (grains, beans, vegetables) than those on the top (fats and sweets). This diet will help keep your heart and body systems healthy.

Another method, similar to the new "plate" USDA food guide, encourages larger portions of vegetables (half the plate) and moderate portions of protein (one-quarter of the plate) and starch (one-quarter of the plate).

Go to this website to get full info on what you need to know about Eating and Diabetes

www.niddk.nih.gov/health-information/diabetes/overview/what-is-diabetes

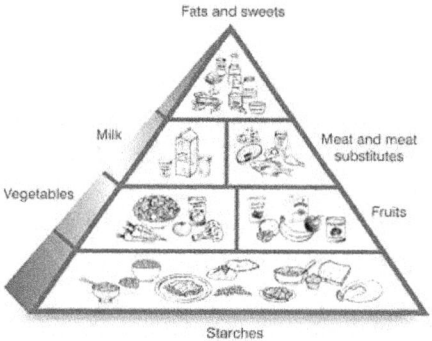

National Institute of Health Food Pyramid

Check out these sites for:

Weight loss:

bit.ly/3zEdEmX

Supports Healthy Circulation:

https://bit.ly/4cQ5HL6

The Sciatica Recovery System +:

https://bit.ly/4cCXE40

Sciatica Recovery. I had a nerve problem when on a trip where I could not get out of bed. I was on a location shoot and lost a full day of filming watching the costs go up and up.

In a way, this is kind of a good thing. If someone is motivated to lose weight and change their direction in their health, they've got a ton of wonderful information at their fingertips.

If you're not a nutrition and exercise expert yourself, how are you supposed to differentiate the good from the bad?

Sample Recipes - Eat Great and Lose Weight

Breakfast Burritos

Ingredients
1-2 tbsp butter
½ cup onion, chopped
2-3 eggs
1 small tomato (preferably Roma), chopped
1-2 tbsp fresh herbs (thyme, rosemary...), minced
2 tbsp soy sauce (wheat free preferably)
¼ cup chopped walnuts or pecans
2-3 tbsp grated raw cheese (optional)
Sprouted Whole Grain (SWG) tortilla

Directions
Heat the butter, add onion, and sauté for 3-4 minutes, stirring frequently.
Scramble the eggs. Add eggs to onions.
Cook for 2 minutes; add tomato, soy sauce, and herbs; and heat until warm.
Stir in walnuts and optional cheese and remove from stove.
Place half of mixture in a line in the center of each SWG tortilla, leaving 1 inch at either end of the line.
Fold each end up to the filling and then fold in one side. Roll.

Viola your breakfast burritos!
Notes you can leave out the tomato and/or walnuts and/or add other veggies... pretty much whatever you like!

If you don't have any tortillas, you can just serve the filling with some sprouted grain toast or some raw veggies.

Mini Vegetable Frittatas

Ingredients

8 large organic eggs
½ cup organic milk, preferably raw
1 Tbsp. butter
1 cup zucchini, diced
1 cup red pepper diced
1 cup sliced fresh mushrooms
1 leek diced
¼ cup fresh Italian flat leaf parsley, chopped finely
1 tsp. Celtic Sea Salt
½ tsp. black pepper

Directions

Preheat oven to 350 degrees F. Grease a large muffin tin with butter. Whisk eggs and milk together in a large mixing bowl. Set aside. Heat butter in a medium skillet or frying pan over medium heat. Place zucchini, red pepper, mushrooms and leek in a skillet and sauté until vegetables become soft, about 5 minutes.

Remove from heat and stir in parsley, salt and pepper. Fold vegetables into egg mixture. Fill muffin cups three-quarters of the way full of vegetable frittata batter. Bake 20 to 30 minutes until frittatas are set and browned on top. Serve hot or cool and store in the fridge for later.

Healthy French toast

Ingredients
2 slices of sprouted grain, rice or spelt bread
2 eggs
1 tablespoon of real butter, maple syrup,
cinnamon

Directions
Mix the eggs in a bowl.
Dip the bread in the egg mixture and
generously coat both sides.

Heat a pan on a low to medium setting and add
the butter.

After the butter melts, add the coated bread.
Cook the bread for 3 to 4 minutes on each side.

Top with cinnamon and maple syrup.

Mediterranean Roast Turkey

(Andrea, a DSP member)

Ingredients

1 large, chopped onion
2 tablespoons freshly squeezed lemon juice
1/2 cup pitted and copped Kalamata olives
1 1/2 teaspoon minced garlic (bottled)
1/2 cup of julienne-cut, oil-packed, sun-dried
tomato halves (drained)
1/2 teaspoon sea salt
3 tablespoons arrowroot powder
1 teaspoon Greek seasoning mix
1 trimmed, boneless turkey breast
1/2 cup fat-free, low-sodium chicken broth
1/4 teaspoon freshly ground black pepper

Directions

Combine turkey, onion, lemon juice, garlic,
tomatoes, sea salt, seasoning mix, olives and
pepper in a crock pot.
Pour in 1/4 cup of chicken broth and let the
ingredients cook for 7 hours.
Combine the arrowroot and the rest of the
chicken broth in a small bowl and whisk until it's
smooth.
Add the mixture to the crock pot. Cover the pot
and cook on low for 30 more minutes.
Slice the Turkey breast after it's cooked.

Exercise and Diabetes:

Healthy Diet Along with Exercise Will Produce Long-term Positive Results

Most diets are considered "fad diets" for a reason. They don't stick around because they are just not realistic for long-term use. I mean c'mon. How long do you think you'll be able to adhere to a juice only diet? Even if you do manage to shed a few pounds, more often than not, you'll gain weight back.

We won't even discuss the nutritional deficiencies you may face when you follow diets that prohibit (or severely limit) carbohydrates, fats, and other essential foods. Your health is your most precious asset. Protect it at all costs. Following a healthy eating plan is the best way to enjoy permanent weight loss results without sacrificing your health.

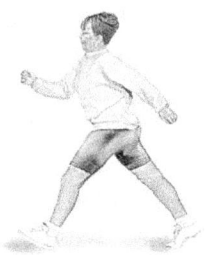

Exercise and A Gym

Anytime a person comes to me and says, will joining a gym help me meet my goals? I simply tell them that no two people are alike. It's all about what works for you. There are a lot of good reasons to join a gym.

Reasons You May Want to Join a gym

- **Motivation.** Everyone at the gym is there for one reason—to exercise. Being around people who share the same goal can motivate you to dig your heels in and get your workouts done. If going to the gym urges you to exercise regularly, then I say go for it!

- **Distractions at Home.** There is always something to do or someone who needs you at home. These distractions can easily take priority (in your mind) over exercising. When you do most of your workouts at the gym, the dishes, dinner, phone calls, laundry and anything else you "need" to do will just have to wait.

- **Access to Exercise Equipment and Fitness Classes.** You don't need much exercise equipment to get a good workout. However, doing the same old exercise videos and running on the same old treadmill can bore you to pieces.

When you opt to work out in a gym, you have access to tons of equipment and a variety of fitness classes, so you rarely get bored.

Gyms like the one I use, Genesis Health Club, are covered on my Medicare Insurance list. Yes, it is true; my **Medicare Advantage plan has a "Gym Membership"** for free because in the long run, it is a smart way to reduce the insurance company's costs by having more healthy people insured. Finally, the idea of preventive health is taking hold over treatment of health problems.

I suggest that you check your healthcare plan; you might find an unexpected surprise membership.

I took the list of gyms in town and looked for the facilities that had what I wanted nearest to my home. I went to Genesis, and it was beautiful, with new equipment and friendly staff.

After working with a "Personal Trainer", I set in on a training meeting with all of their Personal Trainers discussing the topic of "Diabetes and Exercise".

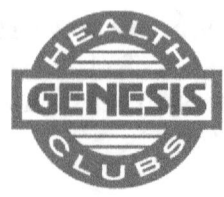

It is very important that your personal trainer knows that you have diabetes so that he or she can adjust your exercise programs for the best results. The following are some notes on what I learned at the meeting.

Key Points:

- Exercise has an insulin-like effect.
- Increased insulin sensitivity due to reducing the need for pancreatic insulin.
- Promotes the utilization and breakdown of blood glucose
- Post-workout glycogen depletion prompts glucose uptake.
- Developing muscles store greater quantities of glycogen.

How to minimize risks & maximize benefits:

- Should have a complete medical evaluation from doctor if exercise is approved.
- Avoid high-impact activities
- Exercise 1 to 3 hours after meals.

- Avoid exercise during peak insulin activity.
- Carry fast acting carbohydrate
- Encouraged to exercise with partner
- Check your feet before and after exercise.

Training Type 2 diabetics:

- American Diabetes Association recommends 1 hour of activity a day.
- Intensity: 40% to 60% of max HR (heart rate)
- Time 30 to 60 min.
- Type: based on tolerance although in people with neurological problems or obese, consider non-weight bearing or resistance training.

Contraindications with Exercise:

- Complications involving retinopathy (Eye Condition)
- High resting blood sugar (>250-300mg/dl)
- Timing not to fall at peak medication activity (+1.5 – 2.5 hours after Insulin)
- Watch for drop in blood pressure with exertion
- Watch for low resting blood sugar (<100 mg/dl) hypoglycemic.

Hypoglycemia:

- Low blood sugar. (**Warning**) Blood sugar under 50 means you have to hold there or higher.
- Symptoms include sweating, nausea, confusion, dizziness, hunger and weakness.
- Treatment: fast-acting carbohydrates such as orange juice or honey followed with a protein source within 20 min of starting episode.
- <u>Not sure</u>, but if it goes down to 'o' you are dead.

Hyperglycemia:

- High blood sugar.
- Symptoms: increased thirst, increased urination, tiredness/drowsiness, headache, blurred vision, dry mouth and/or skin itching.

As more people become diabetic, trainers need to be aware of and how to treat problems because they are in a unique position to help someone in trouble with a problem.

All diabetics are encouraged to exercise with their partner.

Conclusion:

If you have Diabetes type 2, you may have it for life. There are 57 million people who have pre-diabetes, and 1.6 million new cases of diabetes are diagnosed in people aged 20 years or older **each year**.

You can control diabetes by knowing these health facts.

- **Obese**: The number one cause of type 2 diabetes can be controlled by the food you eat.
- **Lack of exercise**: Just make a concerted effort to move around lots more.
- Change your lifestyle to a healthier one.

Changing your life is not hard & none of this is "Rocket Science". Your other option is living 10 years less and in pain with complications of blood sugar that are out of control.

What are Alzheimer's risk factors in 2025 and beyond?

https://my.clevelandclinic.org/health/diseases/9164-alzheimers-disease

Memory:
Memory loss is the most common **A**lzheimer's **D**isease symptom. It can affect your ability to recall recent events (short-term memory) or things that happened a long time ago (long-term memory).
You may have trouble remembering:
   Faces or names
   Facts
   Where you are (even in familiar places like at home)

Memory issues from AD are different and more serious than occasionally forgetting where you left your phone or wondering if you locked the door when you came home.
Researchers don't know why some people get Alzheimer's disease and others don't. Some risk factors may include:
   Being Black or Latino
   Environmental factors (something about where you live, work or spend a lot of time)
   Genetic changes
   Having a traumatic brain injury
   Smoking
   Your age (AD usually affects people older than 65)

Your overall health Some health conditions may increase your Alzheimer's risk, including:
    Cardiovascular disease
    Diabetes
    Down syndrome caused by birth defect
    High blood pressure
    High cholesterol
    Obesity

Complications can include:
    An overall decline in physical health
    Infections (like pneumonia or skin infections)
    Seizures
    Trouble breathing
    Trouble swallowing

You may lose your ability to control your body. This can increase your risk of:
    Bedsores
    Dehydration or malnutrition
    Falls, bone fractures and other traumatic injuries
    Losing control of your pee (urinary incontinence) and poop (bowel incontinence)
    Tooth decay, cavities and other dental issues

In Trials now. To me, and I am not a doctor, it can be summed up by loss of blood flow that allows parts of your brain to malfunction or die. A video I watched talks about blood flow and one of the parts of your blood. *Nitric Oxide* seems to keep your blood vessels in better shape as you get older, which would then seem to slow down or prevent some of these health problems. We seem to be getting close to how to cure some causes of Alzheimer's and maybe even Diabetes 2. Recommended Link for N1O1:

https://bit.ly/4m6qCxq

One more item that seems to be common to later stage Diabetes is Depression:

The relationship between mental depression and diabetes is bidirectional and multifaceted, involving behavioral, biological, psychological, and social mechanisms. Here's a structured overview of their interplay:

1. Directional Relationships
Diabetes Leading to Depression:
Chronic Stress: The daily burden of diabetes management (e.g., blood sugar monitoring, dietary restrictions) can lead to burnout and depressive symptoms.
Physical Complications: Chronic pain, fatigue, or neuropathy from diabetes may reduce quality of life, contributing to depression.
Biochemical Factors: Hyperglycemia and insulin resistance may directly affect brain function, altering mood-regulating neurotransmitters.

Depression Leading to Diabetes:
Behavioral Risks: Depression is linked to poor diet, physical inactivity, and smoking, increasing Type 2 diabetes risk.

Physiological Changes: Chronic stress from depression elevates cortisol, promoting insulin resistance and visceral fat accumulation.

2. Shared Biological Pathways
Inflammation:
Both conditions are associated with elevated pro-inflammatory cytokines (e.g., IL-6, TNF-I±), which may impair insulin signaling and neural function.
HPA Axis Dysregulation: Over activation of the stress response system in depression disrupts glucose metabolism and insulin sensitivity.
Neurotransmitter Imbalances: Serotonin and or epinephrine imbalances in depression may influence appetite dysregulation and glucose homeostasis.

3. Medication Interactions
Antidepressants: Some (e.g., SSRIs, TCAs) can cause weight gain or metabolic changes, increasing diabetes risk.
Diabetes Medications: Certain drugs (e.g., insulin, corticosteroids) may affect mood, though evidence is less clear.

4. Psychosocial and Behavioral Factors
Healthcare Adherence: Depression reduces self-care behaviors (e.g., medication adherence, exercise), worsening glycemic control.
Socioeconomic Factors: Low socioeconomic status exacerbates barriers to

healthcare, healthy food, and safe environments, raising risk for both conditions.

5. Overlapping Symptoms and Diagnosis Challenges:
Symptoms like fatigue, weight changes, and sleep disturbances overlap, complicating diagnosis and treatment.

6. Treatment Implications:
Integrated Care: Addressing both conditions simultaneously improves outcomes. Cognitive-behavioral therapy (CBT) and antidepressants (e.g., SSRIs) may enhance diabetes management.
Lifestyle Interventions: Exercise and dietary changes benefit glycemic control and mood.

7. Complications and Prognosis:
Worse Outcomes: Coexisting depression and diabetes correlate with higher risks of cardiovascular disease, retinopathy, and mortality.
Vicious Cycle: Poor diabetes control exacerbates depression, and vice versa.

8. Statistics and Evidence:
Prevalence: People with diabetes are 2-3 times more likely to experience depression. Conversely, depression increases Type 2 diabetes risk by 60%.

Intervention Studies: Treating depression in diabetic patients often leads to improved HbA1c levels and quality of life.

Conclusion

The interplay between depression and diabetes is complex, involving overlapping biological pathways, behavioral feedback loops, and psychosocial stressors. Effective management requires a holistic approach, integrating mental health care with diabetes treatment to *break the cycle and improve overall health outcomes.*

Remember to ask your doctor about getting a **Constant Blood Monitor**, they are great, and no more sticking your finger over and over.

If this book helped your understanding of Type 2 Diabetes, please post a Review.

Diabetes is not life ending, but you need to think of it often to apply and keep track of it and try not to make things worse.

Thanks,

May this book help someone you love.

Resources

The resources for this book are mostly from the National Institute of Health.

https://bit.ly/4jjvFc4

The American Diabetes Association.

Genesis Health Club

I want to thank all my friends at **Genesis Health Clubs** for all their help in defining exercise programs for the diabetic. Thanks Preston Petersen and John Mc Comb.

Family Health Center Derby, Kansas

I want to thank all my doctors at the **Family Health Center Derby Kansas** for checking and providing the inspiration to write a book to help all type 2 diabetics understand more about their condition and how to make their life better by learning how to combat the condition. Thanks to DR. Mark VinZant and Deborah Benning.

Other Books:

Fly for Free: A Collection of Air Travel tips and Travel Reference guide by Emily Kim)

How to Make Good Photos: Film and Digital Guide

Challenges of an Aircraft Photographer

Flow Posing: A Practical Guide for Wedding Photographers

Wedding Disasters

Blood Harvest: The Entourage (Fiction)

Data Corp: The End of the World (Fiction)

The Secret of Sleepersville 6 (Sci-Fi story written by a friend of mine)

Amazon Author Central

Richard Young Bio is at:
https://amzn.to/44Cciqf

www.ingramcontent.com/pod-product-compliance
Lightning Source LLC
Chambersburg PA
CBHW070613290526
45790CB00002B/891